IF YOU READ THIS, EVERYTHING IS FINE

DAVID MATTAY

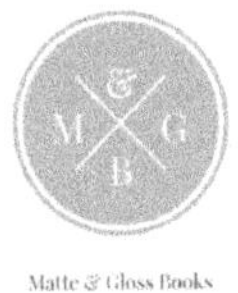

Matte & Gloss Books

Matte & Gloss
books
NO EXTRAWORDYNARY WORKS EXTRAORDINAIRE

EDITURA METRO

Published by Matte & Gloss Books, a non-fiction division of Editura Metro.

First edition: 2021

IF YOU READ THIS, EVERYTHING IS FINE

Cover design: Benjamin Josif

Print ISBN: 978-606-93128-4-1

Ebook ISBN: 978-606-93128-5-8

EDITURA METRO IS AN IMPRINT OF METRO PUBLISHING GROUP.

For Ella.

Without you, this wouldn't exist.

This, and everything else in between.

CONTENTS

INTRODUCTION

I should have been dead now.

By my very own hand.

Instead, I'm trying to find the right words to introduce the pages I wrote then. The day I decided to end my life.

It was a glorious gloomy day. Miserable mournful day. Right in tune with my spirit. I sat at my desk, facing the window. I took out a blank white paper from the drawer.

I had to write a few words to my family. I had to. Not to explain my gesture, no. That is utterly futile. Just to say "Hey, I know I'm a jerk, but look, my last thoughts went towards you."

I sat there, staring at that piece of paper. Maybe for an hour, maybe more. But there were no thoughts. Nada. My mind was blank. Perhaps my brain was too scared to form even a single thought. Dead neurons. Flaccid synapses.

Have you ever been on the high seas? If the weather is good, you could see nothing but infinite waters around you. For miles and miles, not a living soul. But then, out of the blue, something vague appears on the horizon. Another ship? Or it's just Mother Nature mocking you? You can't tell until it is getting closer.

In my case, it was a word. It was naked. And lonely. And meaningless.

IF.

IF?

IF what? IF how? IF why?

I stood there, chewing it. Over and over again. With nothing but emptiness inside.

Men are funny animals. Give them enough time, and they'll make sense of the most improbable things.

And I did have plenty of time. I still have to hear about someone rushing it when they're about to take their own life.

I don't remember exactly how it happened. Maybe at once. Maybe in small increments. But I found myself scribbling furiously. Not the goodbye letter for my family, no. Quite the opposite. Pages after pages of reasons why every life is worth living, no matter what it throws at you.

Far from me thinking that I'm the ultimate holder of the truth. Or the bearer of the key to wisdom and spiritual life. Or the latest guru Illuminati in positive thinking, happiness, and the deep meaning of life.

My only hope is that maybe sometime, somewhere, a wandering, despairing soul will find a spark in here. A foothold in the abyss.

For me, it all started with an IF.

IF YOU HATE YOURSELF, EVERYBODY ELSE WILL, EVENTUALLY

HAVING A BRAIN LARGER THAN OTHER primates is both a blessing and a curse. The marvels of man's world are staggering. So are their hiccups.

Mankind sent men into space. Men walked on the Moon. Machines are flying in deep space right now, beyond the limits of our Solar System. A robot has taken selfies on Mars and then shared them online with billions of people. We sent a space probe that landed on a comet.

And I've listed here only the very tip of the iceberg that humanity is. I've left out mundane things such as instant connection with everybody in the world. Or the fact that the whole human knowledge is - literally! - at one's fingertips. Or the quasi-eradication of ailments that used to take millions of lives, especially those of newborns.

But then, there is hate. And discriminations against. And prejudices. And conflicts. And bloody wars. As if this Blue Pale Dot, this speck we call home in the immensity of the universe (as Carl Sagan famously put it), would not be enough for everyone. As if all the religions and philosophies on Earth would only preach the precepts of the dark forces. Hate thy neighbor. Abhor thy neighbor. Kill thy neighbor.

Or take the tremendous impact we had on our environment since the industrial revolution began 250 years ago. Global warming might be the only modern hoax that would make an entire nation (Maldives) disappear from the face of Earth by the end of this century.

All of these blessings and curses could be traced back to a single thing: the way people look at themselves in the mirror. Friend or foe? "Know thyself", sure and fine, by all means. But how about "Love thyself"?

Imagine our planet hit by a flare from the Sun that would magically make every living soul truly love themselves. In 24 hours, Earth will be the former name of the planet Eden.

Wouldn't the number of narcissists increase exponentially this way? You bet! Though it wouldn't matter. True narcissists are much too absorbed into themselves anyway to make a real difference. But for the rest of the 7-billion-minus-something people, it would make a huge one. Think about it, not only to be at peace with yourself but TO LOVE who you are? And this being the case for every soul out there?

Um, yeah, but the Love Star? And the Love Beam?

It sounds cheesy, I know. But this is not something like "pigs wanting to fly like birds" kind of thing. Nothing is deeming physically impossible for love. It's one of the special powers that everybody has built-in. Much like the eyesight. You were born with the ability to see at a distance that keeps you out of trouble just in case something nasty appears on the horizon. It's the same with the capacity of loving yourself.

It's there. You just have to use it. You have to tickle its button. It will jump from off to on.

Look at the alternatives. Where there's no love, there's indifference at best. But the truth is that nothing stays too long in a no man's land. It will take sides rather sooner than later. Especially when the two most powerful feelings known to man - love and hate - are at stake. In other words, if that inner space of yours is not filled with love, hate is what you're going to milk out of there.

And I'm not talking here about the utterly ugly manifestations of the hate. You don't have to physically - or visibly - hurt other people. Hate is not only hideous but also insidious. It often works in subtle ways, such as despising new things because they are somehow different than what you're used to. And little of this now, a little of that later, one soul poisoned with hate here, a few other millions around, and bam! The world we live in today.

But having love inside? What a tremendous difference this would make! The love inside you would project to the outer world nothing but contentment. Have you ever noticed how you tend to get close to certain people in your life when you feel down? Or, the other way around, in the days when you feel like being on top of the world, how you seem to attract a bunch of people looking for help? It's the same with being filled with love. It affects positively everybody around you.

IF there's one thing you have to stick with after you finish reading this, let it be this: love yourself.

IF YOU FEEL MISUNDERSTOOD, YOU NEED AN INTERPRETER

We've all been there. You struggle to tie a loosely hanging branch of a tree when suddenly you hear a voice behind you saying "Pops, what is that man doing there?" and another one responding "That stupid man is ripping some branches from the nice tree." And you instantly start to feel like Tarzan.

But you know what? Since nobody but yourself is walking in your shoes, how on earth are the other people supposed to know what are you doing or what are you thinking? They have their own problems. They have their own shoes to fill. So you must help them out to understand you. By bringing on the qualified aides.

Ideally, anyone having this kind of problem should be able to hire an interpreter. Do you remember from the history lessons how kings used to have on their payroll a person whose job was to taste the food and drinks before they touched the lips of His Royal Highness? You know, to make sure the king is not poisoned by a very dear friend of his. Mutatis mutandis, what if anyone could have their very own interpreter to help them translate the precise meaning of an action or a speech or a dialogue? "What Mrs. Smith meant was..." "The non-combat attitude of Mr. Smith in yesterday's game must be understood as..." "Ms. Smith was trying to make the point that..."

Maybe in twenty, fifty, or a hundred years from now, when the man will become a cyborg (half-human, half AI), this kind of arrangement would be part of the initial setup. But until then, since the vast majority of people can't even afford to hire themselves, we have to take the next best thing. To work with the interpreters we already have.

There are only two ways in which humans convey messages to each other when they interact. Language and actions.

Language is what you say.

Actions are what you do or what you chose not to do. I know that technically the latter is inaction, but for the sake of simplicity, I'm considering the restraint from doing something an action too.

Language and action are the two interpreters you employ to tell stuff to the other people around you.

IF you feel misunderstood, it's time to revise how they perform. Think and speak in another language (it also helps with decision making). Revamp your actions (body language, what you chose to do, and what you chose not to do).

IF YOU THINK THERE'S NO WAY OUT, YOU NEED A NEW PAIR OF GLASSES

ONLY DEATH IS DEFINITIVE. AND PROBABLY for the majority of Earth's population, even this affirmation is debatable. Everything else is negotiable.

Funny though how so many other instances look as definitive as death does. You don't like your job (or your boss), but you can't quit because the market is bad and the mortgage kicks in every month. You are unhappy in your marriage, but you won't get a divorce because of the kids. You doubled in weight since college, but you can't slim down because you had knee surgery 10 years ago.

Two people can argue to infinity and beyond how a wall is either blue or green. And you know what? Not only they are both right, but the wall is snow white.

Everything there is it's in your head. Every do and every don't. Every can and every can't. It is you and you only who chose how you look at things. The whole world around you and the whole world inside you is a giant kaleidoscope.

IF you think you're at a dead-end, facing a wall so large you can't see its edges, you just have to put on another pair of glasses. And another. And another. Until you find the right one.

IF IT'S THERE, YOU'LL GET IT

One cent.

One cent for every person I had met who stressed the hell out of their socks if I have had, I would have been richer than Croesus by now. And I'm using "stress" here loosely; you can replace it with whatever describes your floundering - struggle, torment, agony, you name it.

So much energy burned for nothing! The energy that otherwise would have found a better use in getting quicker (better, cheaper, etc.) the object of stress. Because in the end, none of this (you, writhing like a demented puppeteer) matters. Either you are stressed out or not, the result will always be the same: if the object of your desire is out there, you will get it. As simple as that.

Of course, you have to be on the path of getting it. You wouldn't want to be in the position of that guy who prayed day and night to the Lord to win the lottery, until one day the Lord himself responded him "Hey buddy, I hear you loud and clear, but how about you buy a lottery ticket for starters, huh?"

I mean, if you want to navigate around the world in a boat that you designed and made, a good idea would be to not live your entire life in the middle of nowhere where you see water only when it rains. How about moving close to the shore, near some people who know how the boats are built?

IF the object of your desire is somewhere out there, just relax. It will be yours.

IF IT'S NOT THERE, YOU EITHER MAKE IT YOURSELF OR WAIT FOR SOMEONE ELSE TO MAKE IT

SOMETIMES WHAT YOU WISH FOR DOESN'T exist yet. Say, immortality. Or traveling to other planets. Or getting fit without moving a finger.

To avoid frustration, there are two ways you can deal with these kinds of wishes: you either work your way up to them, or you sit on your butt and patiently wait for others to make it happen. But getting sour because there aren't any grapes on the other side of the fence? No, no, and no.

If you don't lack resources - any combination of two from these three will do: time, knowledge, and money - probably the best approach is to set things in motion yourself. Yes, somewhere in the world someone bearing the same burn as you might appear, but why lose precious time if you do have what it takes? Start digging around. Do the work. Go find and hire people that might help you either with getting what you want or with getting it quicker.

Everything you use in your daily life (except for maybe a very few serendipitous accidents) appeared because at one point in time somebody wanted it badly. You too could be one of them.

But besides the prospective fame and fortune coming from such an endeavor, let's not forget the giddiest result of them all: the fact that you have put something new in the world. Something that never existed before, but of which - albeit potentially - millions of people can't live without anymore.

IF YOU DON'T GET IT, IT'S BECAUSE THERE'S SOMETHING EVEN BETTER OUT THERE

SOMETIMES IT MIGHT BE YOUR LIFE. How many people were frustrated that they didn't get an invite to a super-duper important meeting held in one of the Twin Towers on the morning of 9/11? Only to see the towers collapse a few hours later? Or, you know, being Seth MacFarlane, oversleeping because of a hangover, getting to the airport 10 minutes after the gates closed, and missing the plane. The American Airlines Flight 11 plane.

IF you are on the path, you are doing your best (80% is showing up, don't forget), but you still don't get that special thing, it might be because along the way there is something better for you. Why settle for less then?

IF IT'S ALL DARK, YOU'LL HAVE TO WAIT FOR THE LIGHT

You see nothing. Not even a slight flicker of a distant star. It's complete darkness. You're wrapped in an opaque, thick texture. Everything has fallen around you. You're lost in space. And there's no fulcrum.

Don't look for the exit button just yet. That button is always there. And unless you become jello overnight, nobody can take it from you. Because here's the thing: this "there's nothing but darkness out there" could be the best thing that happened to you.

But first and foremost, consider this: according to the World Health Organization, the average life expectancy of people on Earth is 73 years. That's about 26,650 sunrises. But even 2,500 years ago, when the life expectancy was less than half that (about 30 years), a man would live to see about 11.000 sunrises. Both figures are large enough to tell us that in the human lifetime, light coming is not an accident. It happens very often. Compare this with mayflies - they only see the light of the sun once. Or with the lifespan of some little beings for which we all should have tremendous respect: the bees. They see the sun's light only about 30 times in their lifetime.

So, for you and me, the light will come rather sooner than later. We don't have to fret if there's complete darkness around us. We just have to sit tight and wait a bit.

Though remember, this darkness could be the best thing that happened to you. Because if it's nothing to see out there, there's a lot to see inside you. I'm amazed how people forget there is always a bare minimum of two universes: the one outside us and the one inside us (sometimes those two collide, but that's another story altogether). And as long as there's a pulse in your veins, there will always be stuff to do about your interior design.

IF IT'S SMALLER, IT WILL GROW

Now, how many times in your life have you looked at something and thought - or said out loud - "Gosh, how small this is!". With a condescending tone, not a dainty one. Regarding your apartment or your bathroom. Your car or your savings account. Your steak or your paycheck.

This ill obsession with big - bigger - biggest drains so much energy out of our lives. Instead of people concentrating on truly important issues. How about ending poverty for good? Or secure access to clean water (and toilets!) for every living soul on Earth?

You don't need a bigger TV screen. A larger house. A shinier smartphone. A faster car. In fact, regarding the material possessions, you need lesser and lesser. Egyptian pharaohs are dead for thousands of years. You aren't one of them, so you can't be buried with your possessions. Okay, if you live in one of the weirder (and less regulated or more corrupted) countries out there, maybe you can. But in either case, you couldn't possibly be a match for Cheops. Why bother?

What truly matters is what you know. And what you know to do. Because these are the only two areas where you can put your dent in the world. Not in how much stuff you got (money, acres, shares, companies, houses, goods, whatever), but in how much knowledge you amassed.

And knowledge, my friend, is like a plant. Every baobab or giant sequoia started as a tiny seed. No matter how little do you know of this or that, given enough time and the right nurture, it will grow.

IF YOU DON'T FIND A REASON, YOU'RE LOOKING IN THE WRONG PLACE

EVERYONE NEEDS A REASON, EVEN LITTLE children. No wonder "why?" is by far the most frequent word in their vocabulary soon after they start talking. And, by the way, "because I said so" is a statement, not a reason.

Do you know who else has reasons? Clinically insane people. Of course, theirs might look like no reasons at all for the others, or they may be utterly illogical, but in their own world and system of references, mad people do have reasons for their actions.

Naturalists have known this principle for a long time: everything in nature happens or is for a reason. (Though I have yet to find a convincing explanation for the existence of mosquitos and flies.) There is a reason behind anything that exists.

Your existence has a reason, too. It might not be apparent for a long time - or ever! - but a reason exists nevertheless.

There are a few fascinating studies on identical twins that show how two human beings, although genetically identical, can have two wildly different lives when separated at birth. One raised Jewish while the other joined the Nazis - that kind of wildness.

Think about it just for a moment. Is it as if two identical balls that start rolling at the same time, in the same spot, and in the same direction, will end up in different places: one at the North Pole and the other at the South Pole. Identical inputs, but so different outcomes. Why? Because each one has its own raison d'être.

So, next time when you just don't understand the reason why something is or isn't, know that you don't see it because you're not looking in the right place. But with enough patience, it will come.

IF THE GLASS IS HALF EMPTY, IT IS BECAUSE YOU DIDN'T FINISH TO POUR

THE EASIEST THING IN LIFE? TO BLAME everything around for whatever happens to you. Your parents. Your siblings. Your village, small town, or big city. The schools and the teachers. The politicians. The rich people. The system. The universe.

But the damn right truth is that you're not a victim. You are what you are and you are where you are because of you and of you only. You have everything - and I mean everything - for making yourself the life you want. To be the person you want to be.

There has never been a better time to be alive in the entire history of humanity. Mute for a few moments the noise coming from the outside world - terrorists, wars, obesity, and so on - and think about it.

You have access to the best education in the world - mostly free or at very low fees - right in front of your big or small screen. You can set up an online business in a matter of minutes. You can sell digital goods to people in over 200 countries and territories without even having a bank account. You can access audiences of billions of people with a few clicks or screen touches. You can have your very own TV show or you can live broadcast whatever happens to you. You can have your own school where you can teach anyone interested in your specific talents or skills.

You are living in a world where you can do anything. And this idea is so important, is worth it to be repeated: you can do anything.

You.

Can do.

Anything.

Be aware. Learn every day. Don't you dare give up. Keep pouring into the glass. One day it will get full.

IF EASY WILL COME, EASY WILL GO

99 OUT OF 100 WINNERS OF LOTTERY jackpots end up much worse than they were before hitting big. And bankruptcy is the lightest of the outcomes. Many of these people pay the highest price of them all for this dramatic shift - with their lives.

Why is this? For one, because is very hard, almost impossible, to cope psychologically with such an event. It is as if a fisherman living at sea level for his entire life would be suddenly transplanted on Mount Everest's peak. His lungs, blood, and brain are used with different concentrations of oxygen. His body is used with different gravitation and outside temperature. Of course that the man is the ultimate adaptability machine - from Eskimos to Tuaregs the man covered all grounds - but this takes time. Hundreds upon hundreds of generations were needed for the man to get closer to the Arctic or deeper into the Sahara desert. Nothing happened in a blink. Nothing happens overnight.

No matter how fluffy it sounds, the truth is that nothing but air comes with the wind. It takes millions and millions of years for the Earth to make a molecule of a diamond. And it takes the same Earth a few nanoseconds to make a molecule of dirt. We all know which of the two elements is the most precious one.

I wouldn't bet against time under any circumstances. Between an extremely talented artist who works only when inspiration strikes and an average talent who puts time and effort into what she or he does, my money is on the latter. Between the turtle that takes one step at a time, slow and steady, and the hasty hare able to run the mile in a blink, on the former.

Paradoxically, but time does equal value even in the eyes of our species. For instance, a single bottle of a 1953 Petrus wine is worth 20 cases of Beaujolais Nouveau, a wine from the crop of the current year. And although most people want to get things or become something with minimal or no effort at all and as quickly as possible, they instinctively look for the oldest person in a group when in need. Though, as the narrative goes, they should be sought for advice (hope, etc.) from a toddler. But somehow only the (very) old age is synonym with wise.

Sand is the easiest construction material known to man. In combination with plain water, it has the ultimate flexibility. You can build virtually anything with sand and water, no matter how complex or simple. Not only that, but you can also do it very quickly and with little to no effort. And both sand and water are abundant in nature. Every ocean, sea, or river on Earth has plenty.

However, not many dwellings are made of sand and water on Earth.

IF YOU NEED HOPE, YOU'LL MAKE IT

HAD MAN LIVED AT THE SAME TIME AS THE dinosaurs, would the dinosaurs still have ruled the Earth? Truck-sized ferocious animals pitted against frail hairless beings, that's a game lost before it begins, right?

Not so fast, Carnotaurus. Though the dinosaurs might have spelled trouble for humans in the beginning, the man would retaliate quickly. Not necessarily because people were so much smarter than the Earth's giants. But mostly because man is the most resilient of the species out there. And the single most important thing that gives us this resilience is hope.

Take hope from the man and you'll get a clod of clay instead. It's such luck then that we were fitted by design with a gland that secrets plenty of this substance of life called hope. A substance so evasive that scientists haven't been able yet to discover the gland that produces it. Though they witnessed and documented its works countless times.

For almost a hundred years communism seemed to be a definitive life sentence for half the Earth's population. Yet people in the affected countries didn't give up hope - as well as those in the free world - and thus today communism is just a parenthesis of history.

Poon Lim, the second steward on the British merchant ship SS Benlomond, thought he was going to die on November 23, 1942, when the German U-Boat U-172 intercepted and sank his ship. SS Benlomond had just left Cape Town, South Africa, a few days before and it was on its way to Paramaribo, Suriname. Though Poon Lim couldn't swim very well, he decided to jump over the board of the rapidly sinking ship. Out of the 54 members of the crew, he was the sole survivor. After the ship had disappeared beneath the ocean, he gasped for air between each wave, desperately looking for a life raft. Finally, after struggling to stay alive for two hours, he found an 8-foot square wooden raft and climbed into it. The raft had several tins of biscuits, a forty-liter jug of water, some chocolate, a bag of sugar lumps, some flares, two smoke pots, and a flashlight. Poon Lim initially kept himself alive by drinking the water and eating the food on the raft, but later resorted to fishing and catching rainwater in a canvas life jacket covering. On April 5, 1943, after 133 days in the raft, he saw a small sail on the horizon, and soon the small boat came to his rescue. He was at the mouth of the Amazon River and had crossed the Atlantic.

IF hope is what you need to survive, you'll make it.

IF YOU CAN MAKE ONE PERSON HAPPY, ANYTHING ELSE IN LIFE IS A BONUS

What you chose to show in a paint or a photo sometimes is least important than what you left out of it. But if it is easily understandable why photographers chose to do this kind of framing, it is harder to see the painters' reasons. Unlike a photographer, for a painter, the immediate universe is not an issue. Why won't they paint stuff that's out of this world, then? (I know, I know - Picasso, Dali, Kandinsky, Magritte, Mondrian, etc. - but still, all the surrealists, symbolists or abstractionists have painted stuff from their immediate worlds) The Earth as seen from the other side of the Universe? Sceneries from the outer worlds? The world before the Big Bang?

Here's the thing: no matter how tempting is (at least for artists), this framing of the proximity has a very simple explanation. Between nothing and infinite, there's only one step.

The white space around us is infinite. Nothing will ever fill it. It doesn't matter how many bazillions of "a man loved a woman" books have been written. Another bazillion of a bazillion books on the same subject won't put even the slightest strain on the white space. And that's the trick. You could choose to do nothing - after all, it is infinity, for crying out loud, nothing matters! Or you could choose to do your part as good as you can, one small step at a time - after all, it is infinity, for crying out loud, everything matters!

And the beauty of it is that you aren't alone. You came upon thousands and thousands of people that have done their part before you. In a way, you build on whatever your forerunners have done. And you pave the way for those who will come after you.

This is the power of one. You put something out there. You pay your dues. You do the best you can (otherwise, why doing anything in the first place?). You win some, you lose some. You keep things in balance for as long as you can.

It doesn't matter who you are, what country you are living in, on which side of the IQ scale you find yourself, what is the color of your skin, or how many years you spent in school. There is one thing anyone can do. To take one step. THAT ONE STEP. One step that closes the gap between nothing and infinite. Make one person happy. Even yourself, if this is the best you could come up with. As long as you being happy doesn't make any other living soul unhappy, it's perfectly fine.

IF you can make one person happy, anything else in your life it will come as a bonus.

It doesn't matter who you are. What country you are from, on which side of the [illegible] you find yourself, what is the color of your skin, or [illegible] [illegible] is [illegible] [illegible] THAT ONE SIMPLE [illegible] that does [illegible] nothing [illegible] Make this person happy. Even yourself. [illegible]

[illegible]

IF YOU BELIEVE, THERE YOU HAVE IT

FAITH IS THE STRONGEST WEAPON OF humankind. The strongest medicine. The strongest tool. Nothing can stand against a man of faith.

Faith's enormous power comes from its intrinsic frailty. You believe, therefore you have. You have the power of doing anything. The power of being anything. The power of having everything.

That's the reason why the ways of the faith are paved with blocks. Huge, enormous ones. Men of faith are often derided. Somehow their faith makes them utterly insane in the eyes of other people. Because you know what? Just like an insane person, a man of faith sees things where they aren't.

Copernicus, Boltzmann, Mendel, or Zwicky were all considered loonies by the scientific community of their time. Decades and sometimes hundreds of years had to pass before their ideas were accepted. Yes, you need guts to walk the walk of shame amongst your contemporaries, but guess what? We all know who Copernicus and Mendel were, what did they stand for, and what have they done for the world at large. But can you name a single detractor of these people? Yeah, neither can I.

Believe. And there it is.

IF EVERYTHING IS AN ILLUSION, YOU CAN BE THE GREATEST ILLUSIONIST EVER

So what if everything is an illusion? You say gloom, I say great. If those scientists working their asses off to demonstrate that we're living in a virtual reality are right, so be it. Nothing is real - you, me, this book you're reading, the chair or the sofa you're sitting on. Fine, but why this should bother us? If what's truly real is a virtual reality, not even the sky is the limit. We're living in a limitless world. We just have to learn how to bend this world around us. Like illusionists do.

However, given the scale - the whole world being indeed a scene, as the Bard used to say - why won't we start working on some global illusions? For instance, what if we terminate this nonsense with countries and borders? We're part of the same illusion, so people should be able to roam freely inside this illusory bubble, right? Also, regarding personal wealth: why accumulate wealth as an individual? An illusion is an illusion - I'll show you mine, you'll show me yours, and neither of us can say that one is bigger than the other. So, how about forgetting about this idea of personal wealth and instead gather all the eggs in the same basket? You know, for the greater good of our common illusion. Of course, there are people much more talented than others at making money, and they can still keep score among them. How much illusion they brought to the table, let's say. We can even set up a new Pantheon to praise (and please) them all.

But until we'll figure out what we're going to do on a global level, how about each one of us believe that everything is an illusion to begin acting like this is the case? Let's walk the walk on the path of becoming the greatest illusionist the world has ever seen. Who's first?

IF YOU START WITH THE END IN MIND, BEGINNINGS WILL BE A BREEZE

GROPE & HOPE.

That's what should be written on the forehead of the vast majority of people. We fumble about in life without the slightest idea where do we want to arrive. What do we want to get. To know. To do. To accomplish. Shouldn't the Brownian motion be suited with a name such as the Homo Sapiens motion?

This doesn't mean we need to be stuck with an idea our entire life. We are people, not trains rolling on rails. We can take a turn anytime we want. And yes, we can change the destination as many times as we darn please, thank you very much! But the magic word here is the destination. We better have a precise idea of where we want to go.

Procrastination is a myth. A fancy word to label the aimless move through life. Of course, we won't budge a pinkie if we have no idea for what. Energy is expensive, it goes without saying that we'll save as much as we can.

Next, when you - or someone else, for that matter - beat you up for being lazy and not doing what you're supposed to do, stop for a moment and think if you have a clear goal towards you are going. Because if not, you should work on that in the first place.

Whatever you want to start in life - painting, slimming down, running a marathon, climbing Mount Everest, colonize the planet Mars, etc. - start with the end in mind. What do you want to achieve? What is your ultimate goal? What is at the end of that road?

And you'll never ever encounter again the problem of not doing what you're supposed to do.

IF LIFE IS ALL THAT YOU GOT, YOU GOT EVERYTHING

MOAN AT LENGTH IF YOU LIKE. SHOUT YOUR despair. Or your deepest fears. Cry even, with real tears. Wet things on you. Flood the space around you.

It feels good to let it all out from time to time. It's cathartic. And there is no shame in it.

However.

Nevertheless.

But.

Do not allow this act of internal reset to obfuscate the truth. You are alive. You are breathing.

Shh! Feel it. Hear it.

In.

Out.

I-in.

O-out.

I-i-i-in.

O-o-out.

Good. Now deepen your senses inside you.

Tick-tock! Tick-tock! Tick-tock!

Hello-o-o heart! That's your ticker alright. It makes your eardrums pop out slightly. Which is the perfect illustration of the "alive and kicking" saying.

A wonderful feeling this one, of being alive. Even if you think you're living the biggest tragedy from the ancient Greeks until today, it is still good to be alive. And you know why? Because you have the privilege of thinking you are in the middle of the most tragic events since 500 B.C.

Death is easy. But the beauty is that life is not hard. Life just is.

IF IN DOUBT, CHOSE LOVE

It's no wonder successful people ignore making mundane decisions to concentrate on really important ones. The willpower can be as easily exhausted as the battery of your smartphone. And boy, how modern life throws at us thousands of tiny decisions we have to make!

The explosion of choices after WWII is downright staggering. Where our grandparents had maybe five car models to chose from, we have something like five hundred. Plus at least ten different ways of making the purchase. And don't even start me on something basic such as bread. I bet there are at least a thousand varieties of them on the "no gluten" camp alone.

When people talk about the "simpler life" of the past, they usually have in mind the fewer choices they used to have only a few decades ago.

There are a lot of voices out there saying the rocketing rates of obesity in the past four decades are the result of people eating more and moving less. (Plus the usual culprits, the macronutrients, which came one by one as the greatest villain of the people's waists. Fat, carbohydrate and protein were all burned at the stake one time or another.) But my wild - mild? - guess is that the explosion of obesity came into the world just about at the same time as the explosion of the choices people had in their lives. And hence, the decisions needed to be made daily. When you're confronted with thousands of decisions along the day, there's little surprise that very soon your willpower will be depleted. And that piece of broccoli you know is good for you (after all, your mother told you so!) suddenly looks much less appetizing than an extra-large chocolate bar or a greasy burger served with a pound of fries and a gallon of soft drink.

You too need to reduce the number of decisions you have to make. Put everything you can on autopilot. And spare your willpower to concentrate on the really important issues in life. Because unless you aren't that ideal and perfect figure existing in all human cultures across the globe, you have to have a bunch of them.

How to know if you are going to make the best decisions you can? Easy: whenever you are in doubt, chose love. How is your decision going to affect your significant other? Your children? Your family at large? Your friends? Your colleagues? The community you're living in? Your immediate environment? The Old Blue Planet? Anything can be filtered through these lenses.

You'll know it in your gut if your decision will affect them lovingly or destructively. If you will add something to the table or if you will subtract something. If you will give more than you will take. If the scale leans towards the right way.

Always. Chose. Love.

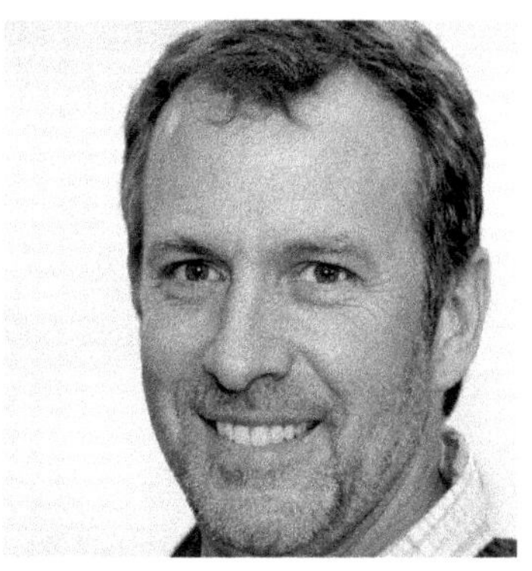

DAVID MATTAY is a trained lawyer who became a composer, following his life-long passion for music and string instruments. When he's not writing music, David tends his garden while trying to learn all the bird calls and songs he can hear. David lives in Europe with his wife, three kids, five dogs, and two cats. Of all the souls living under the same roof, he's the only one who doesn't like fish.

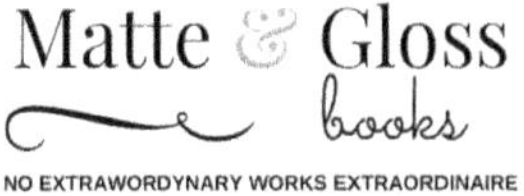

DISCLAIMERS

WARRANTIES DISCLAIMER The authors and publishers don't guarantee or warrant the quality, accuracy, completeness, timeliness, appropriateness, or suitability of the information in this book, or of any product or services referenced by it.

The information in this book is provided on an "as is" basis and the authors and publishers make no representations or warranties of any kind concerning this information. This book may contain inaccuracies, typographical errors, or other errors.

LIABILITY DISCLAIMER The publishers, authors, and any other parties involved in the creation, production, provision of information, or delivery of this book specifically disclaim any responsibility, and shall not be liable for any damages, claims, injuries, losses, liabilities, costs, or obligations including any direct, indirect, special, incidental, or consequential damages (collectively known as "Damages") whatsoever and howsoever caused, arising out of, or in connection with, the use or misuse of the book and the information contained within it, whether such damages arise in contract, tort, negligence, equity, statute law, or by way of any other legal theory.

www.ingramcontent.com/pod-product-compliance
Ingram Content Group UK Ltd.
Pitfield, Milton Keynes, MK11 3LW, UK
UKHW021933190726
13853UKWH00004B/1422

9 786069 312841